Bodybuilding Nutrition: 50 Meals, Snacks and Protein Shakes

Simple Meals to Build Muscle, High Protein Recipes For Getting Ripped, Vegetarian Protein Meals for Muscle Building

By
M Laurence

Table of Contents

34. Snack - Mexican Black Beans and Avocado
35. Snack - Raisin Oatmeal Cookie
36. Snack - Fast Yogurt and Apricot
37. Snack - Protein Banana Smoothie
38. Snack - Guacamole Hummus
39. Snack - Sweet Cinnamon Quinoa Punch
40. Snack - Protein Apple and Celery Smoothie
41. Snack - Peppermint Oatmeal Shake
42. Snack - Iced Breakfast Shake
43. Snack - Almond Blast Shake
44. Snack - The Berry Super Shake
45. Snack - Chocolate and Banana Shake
46. Snack - Chocolate Cherry Shake
47. Snack - Superfood Shake
48. Snack - The Power Shake
49. Snack - Choco Peanut Butter Shake
50. Snack - Mango Shake
Bonus Shake
The Number One Mistake to Avoid!

Rugby Body Optimal Nutrition = Optimal Gains

As we all know building muscle size is a simple combination of hard training and nutrition. Put like that it sounds very easy. To go one step further with nutrition - we must consume more calories than we are burning in a single day - everyday. Otherwise there is no fuel to build additional muscle mass and we will never ever grow size.

Most people know how to workout. Most people know the fundamentals for working each muscle group and allowing rest. However the part most people fall down on is nutrition. This is the first mistake a lot of newbies make when entering the world of muscle building. But not only newbies think they can train harder and still grow even though they aren't consuming enough calories. I've seen many guys who workout for years and make no gains just because they hadn't got their diet plan on point.

Bodybuilding is nutrition and whether you want an extra two inches on your arms or you want to add 25lbs of overall muscle mass it is all about the food you ingest. Improving your workout technique is very important – absolutely and knowing when to rest is also vital in creating the physique you want, but if your nutrition isn't nailed, it will all be for nothing.

So with this book I wanted to create a fast, easy-to-hand reference guide that will work alongside my previous book 'How To Build The Rugby Player Body'. This book contains a full workout and diet plan.

How To Build The Rugby Player Body
Paperback
https://www.createspace.com/6252083

But I wanted more diet options and I wanted it simple. 50 recipes – Breakfasts first, then lunches, dinners and finally snacks which will include a range if protein-heavy shakes.

I wanted to give focus to high protein meals, and more importantly a variety of proteins meals. Lots of simple yet delicious recipes including chicken and beef but more choice such as Tuna burgers, Quorn Lasagne, Salmon salads, Tofu Chilli, and mocha pancakes and many more.

If you're like me then you aren't a fan of consuming chicken and broccoli every day 4 times a day. I need variation when it comes to diet and nutrition and today we have a huge array of protein-packed foods for building muscle at our very finger tips. My training book covered many meat and poultry options so I wanted to not only include these options but look to some other options including vegetarian protein too.

More and more bodybuilders are mixing their beef and nuts and Tofu and Quorn. It's because we can supply a mix of amino acids for our muscles. Varity like varying exercises is great for the body. Plus they do contain a surprising amount of high quality protein and taste great. Gone are the days where veggie foods tasted like catfood.

Now we have an incredible selection, and I intend to use these not only taste variation, but a variation in protein, all good for the body.

So what calories should we be consuming? A mix of protein, carbs and fats. The ratios vary from expert to expert and, but i go for a 40% Protein, 40% Carbs and 20% Fats. These figures can vary body to body. It's up to you to try things out and see how your body reacts.

Not only will you find 50 recipes from breakfast, lunch and dinner, but also protein shakes, snacks and I encourage you to swap out ingredients to get creative.

I'm also forever adding a little healthy punch to post-workout meals:

- Adding more whole or egg whites
- A table spoon of natural Peanut Butter with a shake.
- Three table spoons of Cottage Cheese with lunch
- Handful of Cashew Nuts with a black coffee

Obviously eggs and diary are a great source of protein (if you eat them).

Let's take a look at what exactly high-protein Vegetarian foods are available to utilize in your meals that I include in my recipes.

MYCOPROTEIN (QUORN)
Protein: 13 grams per 1/2 cup serving

SOY
Protein: 10 grams per 1/2 cup serving (firm tofu); 15 grams per 1/2 cup serving (tempeh); 15 grams per 1/2 cup serving (natto)

QUINOA
Protein: 8 grams per 1 cup serving, cooked

BUCKWHEAT
Protein: 6 grams per 1 cup serving, cooked

HEMPSEED
Protein: 10 grams per 2 tablespoon serving

CHIA
Protein: 4 grams per 2 tablespoon serving

EZEKIEL BREAD
Protein: 8 grams per 2 slice serving

SEITAN
Protein: 21 grams per 1/3 cup serving

SPIRULINA WITH GRAINS OR NUTS
Protein: 4 grams per 1 tablespoon

HUMMUS AND PITA
Protein: 7 grams per 1 whole-wheat pita and 2 tablespoons of hummus

PEANUT BUTTER SANDWICH
Protein: 15 grams per 2-slice sandwich with 2 tablespoons of peanut butter

Without further ado let's get to the receipts!

1. Breakfast - Pumpkin Vanilla Oatmeal

This will take 5 minutes and will create a new love for Oatmeal, I swear by this a fantastic pre-workout when I need some heavy-duty energy.

INGREDIENTS

- Rolled oats: 1/2 cup
- Water: 1 cup
- Canned pumpkin: 1/3 cup
- Whey Isolate vanilla protein powder: 1/2 scoop
- Pumpkin pie spice: 1/2 tsp
- Maple syrup: 1 tsp (or sugar-free syrup)
- Chopped pecans: 1 tsp
- Chopped raisins: 1 tsp

DIRECTIONS

In a medium-sized microwave-safe bowl, combine the oats and water. Pop them in the microwave for two minutes. You may need to stir after 1 minute and then put it on again for a further 1 min.

Remove oats from the microwave and stir in the canned pumpkin, protein powder, pumpkin pie spice, and maple syrup. Top with raisins and pecans. Then Enjoy!

Tip - Depending on taste you could add a full protein scoop and to get another 12 grams of protein.

NUTRITION FACTS

Serving size: 1 bowl
Amount per serving

- Calories 298
- Fat 9.4 g
- Carbs 41.9 g
- Protein 16.2 g

2. Breakfast - Mega Eggs and Quinoa

This is a hard-hitting breakfast - packed with a whopping 44grams of protein and a healthy dose of carbs if you have the side dish - ideal before or after a workout or to see you through to Lunch.

INGREDIENTS

- 225g - firm Tofu (chopped or crumbled)
- 3 - Egg Whites
- 1 - Whole Egg
- 2 - cups Spinach
- 1/2 - cup sliced Mushrooms
- 1/2 - cup Cherry Tomatoes
- Olive Oil, fresh Garlic, Soy Sauce, Lemon Juice and Salt and Pepper.

DIRECTIONS

Whisk the egg and egg whites together in a jug.
Add tomatoes, mushrooms, and 1 clove of garlic (crushed or chopped) into warmed frying pan and cook until the mushrooms have softened, turning slightly golden brown.
Add egg mixture to frying pan with tomatoes and mushrooms, stirring occasionally.

Tip - I like to sieve the egg mix as I pour it into the frying pan or saucepan. This removes all the gooey bits haha - try it and see if you approve.

As the scrambled eggs begin to set - Turn the heat to low and add the tofu, a splash of soy sauce, splash of lemon, and your salt and pepper to taste.
Cook letting some of the liquid cook off and the tofu to warm up.

Turn off the heat and mix in the spinach.

NUTRITION FACTS

Serving size: 1 crepe with filling
Amount per serving
- Calories 308
- Fat 14 g
- Carbs 61 g
- Protein 44 g

3. Breakfast - Coconut Vanilla Protein Crepes

These delicious tasting Crepes pack a serious protein blast at 65 grams.

INGREDIENTS: CREPE MIXTURE

- Egg Whites: 4
- Instant Oats: 1/2 Cup
- Ripe Banana: 1
- Whey Isolate Vanilla Protein Powder : 1 Scoop
- Vanilla Extract: 1/2 Tsp

INGREDIENTS: FILLING INGREDIENTS

- Nonfat Greek Yogurt: 1 Cup
- Natural Peanut Butter (Or Met-Rx Powdered Peanut Butter): 2 Tbsp
- Ground Cinnamon: 1/2 Tsp
- Vanilla Extract: 1/2 Tsp
- Honey Or Agave: 1 Tbsp

DIRECTIONS

Put all crepe ingredients in a blender, and mix for 30 seconds. If mixture is too thick, add a tablespoon of water until a smooth, pourable batter consistency is achieved.

Cook crepes in coconut oil for 20 seconds each side in preheated pan.

Fill each crepe with banana and yogurt filling – enjoy!

NUTRITION FACTS

Serving size: 1 crepe with filling

Amount per serving

- Calories 608
- Fat 7.5 g
- Carbs 71 g
- Protein 65 g

4. Breakfast - Cinnamon Quinoa

This is a fantastic variation to Oats and goes down so smoothly. This is just one reason why I love Quinoa.

INGREDIENTS

- 1/4 cup cooked Quinoa
- 1 palm-full of Walnuts or Pecans
- 1 palm-full of Blackberries or Blueberries
- Sprinkle of Cinnamon
- Sweeten with Stevia (zero-calorie natural sweetener) or use agave nectar or some soft Honey.

DIRECTIONS

Cook your Quinoa in a saucepan of boiling for water for 15 minutes (you can add a splash of soy milk, almond milk, or hemp milk if you want it to be moister).
Drain the water from the Quinoa and put into a separate large bowl.
Add the walnuts, blackberries, cinnamon and Stevia and mix it all together with a spoon.

NUTRITION FACTS

Serving Size (including Quinoa on the side)
Amount per serving
- Calories 418
- Total Fat 26g
- Total Carbs 29g
- Protein 44g

5. Breakfast - Grab-N-Go Protein Hit

This is a time-efficient Breakfast - prepare the night before - grab and go in the morning with a heavy duty 22 grams of protein.

INGREDIENTS

- 1/4 - cup Rolled Oats
- 1/2 - cup Almond Milk
- 1/2 - scoop Chocolate Protein Powder
- 1 - Large Spoon of Natural Yogurt
- 1 - Banana
- 1 - tbsp Chia Seeds
- 1/2 - tbsp Cinnamon

DIRECTIONS

Mix all ingredients together in a large bowl - slice banana on top and add more Protein powder and Yogurt if additional protein is needed.
Once finished place in plastic container in fridge overnight.

Grab and go in the morning for a fast start to the day.

The easy thing with this is you can take away the oats if you just want a protein hit and this becomes a mid-morning snack. Add more honey to it to spike insulin levels and it becomes the perfect post workout hit.

NUTRITION FACTS

Recipe serves 1
Amount per serving
- Calories 306
- Total Fat 15.6 g
- Total Carb 32.1 g
- Protein 22.7 g

6. Breakfast - Mocha Pancakes

Coffee Pancakes provide a sure-fire way to rev up your morning workout. The batter can be made the night before and chilled. Whole-wheat pastry flour or spelt flour can be substituted for oat flour.

You can grind up oats into a fine powder which has a denser supply of fibre, vitamins, and minerals than your typical all-purpose flour.

INGREDIENTS

- Oat flour: 3/4 cup
- Plain or vanilla protein powder: 1/4 cup
- Cocoa powder: 2 tbsp
- Cinnamon: 1 tsp
- Baking powder: 1 tsp
- Baking soda: 1/2 tsp
- Large egg: 1
- Strongly brewed coffee (cooled to room temperature): 3/4 cup
- Vanilla extract (omit if using vanilla protein powder): 1 tsp
- Banana, mashed: 1/2 medium
- Hazelnuts or walnuts, chopped: 2 tbsp
- Unsalted butter or coconut oil: 2 tsp
- Raspberries: 1 cup

DIRECTIONS

In a large bowl, stir together the flour, protein powder, cocoa powder, cinnamon, baking powder, baking soda, and a pinch of salt.
In a separate bowl, whisk together the egg, coffee, and vanilla extract. Stir in the mashed banana and nuts.

Add the wet ingredients to the dry ingredients, mix gently, and let the batter rest 15 minutes.
Melt butter or coconut oil in a skillet over medium heat. Pour 1/4 cup batter for each pancake into the pan, and cook for 2 minutes per side.
Serve the pancakes topped with raspberries, and drizzle them with pure maple syrup if desired.

NUTRITION FACTS

Serving Size: 1/2 recipe, about 4 pancakes
Recipe yields: 2 Servings
- Calories: 425
- Fat: 13 g
- Carbs: 50 g (13 g fibre)
- Protein: 28 g

7. Breakfast - Protein-Packed Oatmeal

The classic oatmeal breakfast - easy to prepare - excellent slow carbs 29 grams - big on 23 grams of protein with added powder.

INGREDIENTS

- 1/4 - cup Rolled Oats
- 1/4 - cup berries, choose your preference (I used Blueberries)
- 1/2 - cup water - or Oat Milk, Soya Milk, Coconut Milk - you're choice!
- 1/2 - scoop Protein Powder - choose your preference (I usually go for Vanilla)
- 1 - tbsp all-natural Peanut Butter

DIRECTIONS

Place the berries in a microwave-safe bowl and microwave for 30 seconds.
Remove and smash the berries with a fork.
Add oats, water, and protein powder.
Microwave the mixture for 1.30 minutes - then stir - microwave for another 1 minute.

Stir and top with peanut butter if you want even more protein. Or add more protein powder, but it can become a little thick with too much. Also I've found i have to add more water/milk after the first microwave.

In a Saucepan
This does taste better - Add oats and water/milk and protein powder to a saucepan - stir and heat up until it starts to boil. Then leave it for 5 minutes stirring occasionally. Then reheat and serve.

NUTRITION FACTS

Recipe serves 1
Amount per serving
- Calories 317
- Total Fat 12.7 g
- Total Carb 29.4 g
- Protein 23.6 g

8. Breakfast - Early Riser Breakfast

This breakfast will cook in the oven as you get yourself ready for the day. Perfect after an early morning workout.

INGREDIENTS

- Egg Whites 6
- Asparagus 2-3
- Brown Rice And Quinoa Mix 1/2 Cup
- Red Bell Pepper 1 Sliced
- Garlic, Pepper, And Sea Salt 1 Pinch
- Grapefruit 1/2 Pink
- Dymatize Iso 100 1 Scoop

DIRECTIONS

Set oven to 405 F.
Lightly spray a cast iron skillet with coconut oil or olive oil.
Add cooked brown rice and quinoa to the skillet.
Pour in egg whites, and then add asparagus strips and pieces and bell pepper slices.
Bake in the oven for 15-18 minutes (or until eggs are cooked).

NUTRITION FACTS

Amount per serving
- Calories 407
- Total Fat 2 g
- Total Carb 46 g
- Protein 52 g

9. Breakfast - Muscle Building Pancake

A little more time is required - but very tasty - and at 33 grams of protein and 30 grams of superb carbs it's a great start to the day.

INGREDIENTS

- 6 - Egg Whites
- 1/2 - cup Oats
- 1 - scoop Protein Powder (Any Flavour)
- 1/2 - cup of flour
- 2 - tbsp Sugar-free Pancake syrup

DIRECTIONS

Mix the egg whites, oats, flour and Protein Powder in a jug. Heat a non-stick pan over medium-high heat and coat with 0 cal non-stick spray.
Pour 1/4 cup of the pancake batter into the pan and let cook until bubbles begin to appear. Pour more mixture. Flip and cook on the other sides until firm.
Serve with the syrup.

If you're feeling creative why not add some blue berries to the mix - they taste great!

NUTRITION FACTS

Serving Size: 2
Amount per serving
- Calories 292
- Total Fat 5g
- Total Carbs 30g
- Protein 33g

10. Breakfast - Frittata with Zucchini

Zucchini is a rich source of flavonoids, that harm free radicals, which play a role in the aging process. It is low in calories and contain a wonderful bounty of vitamin C another good antioxidant.

INGREDIENTS

- 3 eggs
- ¼ cup of Parmesan cheese
- ¼ teaspoon Mediterranean Sea salt
- 2 tablespoons olive oil
- 1 clove, minced garlic
- 1 small zucchinis, shredded
- 1 red peppers, cut into strips

DIRECTIONS

Eggs provide the high impact protein and using half the yolks ensure that cholesterol levels are kept in check. Preheat the oven to 400 degrees. In a medium bowl, whisk the first four ingredients. Heat oil in a skillet that can be placed in the oven, add garlic and cook for one minute or until just tender.

Add the zucchini and peppers and cook for another minute. Pour in the egg mixture and cook about three minutes or until the bottom of the mixture is set. Bake in the oven to finish cooking for about ten minutes.

NUTRITION FACTS

Serving Size: 1
Amount per serving
- Calories 332
- Total Fat 9g
- Total Carbs 18g
- Protein 29g

11. Breakfast - Italian Omelet

This Italian omelet is going to provide high protein and high doses of vitamins including C with the bell peppers.

INGREDIENTS

- 1 Tbsp. chopped green bell pepper
- 1 Tbsp. chopped onion
- 1 Tbsp. chopped tomatoes + a little extra for garnish
- 3 eggs, beaten
- 1 tsp Italian seasoning
- 1 tsp fresh Parmesan cheese

DIRECTIONS

Place the egg in the pan, after you have beaten them. Once the egg starts to cook add the vegetables.

NUTRITION FACTS

Serving Size: 1 serving
Amount per serving
- Calories 313
- Total Fat 10g
- Total Carbs 12g
- Protein 23g

12. Lunch - Bagel with Salmon and Cream Cheese

This a fast and simple lunch, on the go, quick to make and put in a bag to eat later. Salmon is not only packed with healthy Protein it also contains heart healthy omega 3-fatty acids.

INGREDIENTS

- Use fat free cream cheese
- 3 Ounces Smoked salmon (17grams of protein)
- Cucumber, sliced
- Tomato sliced
- Leaves of lettuce
- Choice of bagel

DIRECTIONS

Using a choice of bagel, spread 1 Tbsp. of cream cheese on each side of the bagel. Place 3 ounces of salmon on the bagel. Top it will lettuce, cucumber, and tomato. Cut into chunks to easily eat on the go.

NUTRITION

Serving Size: 1 serving
Amount per serving
- Calories 299
- Total Fat 15g
- Total Carbs 33g
- Protein 32g

13. Lunch - The Epic Tortilla

Not for the faint hearted! Will need preparing before work if not at home - an epic lunch of 32 grams of protein.

INGREDIENTS

- 1 - 8 Inch Whole Tortilla
- 1 - Whole Egg
- 3 - Egg Whites
- 1 - Lettuce Leaf
- 2 - tbsp kidney Beans
- 1 - tbsp reduced-fat grated Cheese
- 1/4 - cup Salsa

DIRECTIONS

Lightly coat a medium non-stick frying pan with cooking spray and place over medium heat. Place tortilla in the frying pan and warm for 30 seconds, then flip and warm the other side for 30 seconds. Place the warmed tortilla on a small plate.

Whisk the egg and egg whites together. Pour into the frying pan and cook, stirring occasionally, until set.
Place the lettuce leaf on the tortilla and spread the kidney beans over the lettuce leaf. Top the beans with the cooked eggs, add grated cheddar cheese, and 2 tablespoons of salsa.
Roll it up and top with remaining salsa.

Tip - Why not cut it up into sections and use it as a super snack before and after the gym.

NUTRITION FACTS

Serving Size: 1 serving
Amount per serving
- Calories 313
- Total Fat 10g
- Total Carbs 30g
- Protein 32g

14. Lunch - Tuna with White Bean Salad

Tuna is a fantastic protein choice and so are Vitamin rich tomatoes. Tuck into this ultra-healthy salad.

INGREDIENTS

- 1/3 cup tomato juice
- 3 tablespoons lemon juice
- 2 tablespoons olive oil
- 1 tablespoon fresh basil, chopped or 1 teaspoon dried
- ¼ teaspoon salt
- 1 6-ounce can tuna, drained
- 1 can 15 ounces' white beans, drained and rinsed
- 1 medium cucumber, peeled, seeded and chopped
- ¼ cup pitted Kalamata olives, chopped
- 6 cups of mixed salad greens

DIRECTIONS

In a small bowl, whisk together the first five ingredients. In a medium bowl, toss the next four ingredients with one tablespoon of vinaigrette. Divide the greens among four plates. Top with a quarter of the tuna mixture and drizzle with dressing.

NUTRITION FACTS

Serving Size Per serving, recipe makes 4 servings
Amount per serving
- Calories 241
- Total Fat 12g
- Total Carbs 24g
- Protein 59g

15. Lunch – Pure Protein Lemon Herb Salmon

Leaning up? Try this low-carb high-protein lunch.

INGREDIENTS

- 3 ounces of Salmon
- One lemon
- Ginger
- Garlic
- Celery seeds
- Oregano

DIRECTIONS

Use the herbs to taste. Simply place them over the salmon and squeeze the lemon juice onto the fish. Lay sliced lemon over the salmon, bake it at 350 degrees F until it is cooked. Depending on the thickness of the salmon it may take 10 to 20 minutes.

NUTRITION

Serving Size: 1
Amount per serving
- Calories 190
- Total Fat 12g
- Total Carbs 2g
- Protein 18g

16. Lunch - Chicken Salad with Nuts

Chicken is a healthy food, not only because it is low in cholesterol, but because of its antioxidant properties. Combine it with walnuts and cranberries and you will definitely add healthy components that help your skin.

INGREDIENTS

- 2 Tbsp. mayo
- ½ pound chicken
- 1 Cup Cous Cous
- ¼ cup cranberries
- ¼ cup walnuts

DIRECTIONS

Cook Cous Cous for 10 mins on a pan. Combine the rest of the ingredients in a bowl, with the chicken, diced then - spread the chicken salad over the Cous Cous.

NUTRITION FACTS

Serving Size: 1
Amount per serving
- Calories 230
- Total Fat 15g
- Total Carbs 40g
- Protein 22g

17. Lunch - Broccoli Chicken Stir-fry

Stir-fry is just a way to say you have a lot of vegetables and meat to place over Ramen or Rice. What you put in a stir fry is up to you, but if you want healthy skin, then the suggestions for this recipe will definitely provide antioxidants, plus vitamins C, E, and A. Broccoli is also known to help with skin regeneration and repair due to a property called glucoraphanin.

INGREDIENTS

- 3 Ounces of chicken
- 2 heads of broccoli
- 1 carrot
- 1 cup of seaweed
- Peppers
- Onion
- Water chestnuts
- Bamboo shoots

DIRECTIONS

If there are any vegetables such as mushrooms that you like, you can add them. The main point is to have the broccoli and chicken in the dish. You can decide to use soy sauce or another stir-fry sauce. One with ginger is a good option since ginger also has antioxidant and anti-inflammatory properties. Brown rice is best for health reasons. Simply cook the chicken, add the carrots and other hard vegetables once the chicken is cooked. Add in the sauce and the rest of the vegetables, let cook until the vegetables are cooked and serve over rice or noodles.

NUTRITION FACTS

Serving Size: 1
Amount per serving
- Calories 302
- Total Fat 25g
- Total Carbs 34g
- Protein 35g

18. Lunch - Tuna Burger And Salad

This is a great alternative to eating your tuna that boasts a high protein content and a healthy level of good fat.

INGREDIENTS
- Tuna 1 Can
- Egg Whites 1
- Dry Oats 1/4 Cup
- Organo, Garlic, Onion Powder
- Olive Oil 1 Tbsp
- Mixed Veggies 1/2 Cup
- Romaine Lettuce 2 Cups
- Salad Dressing 2 Tbsp

DIRECTIONS

Mix together the chunk light tuna, egg white, and dry oats and form into a patty.

Heat the oil in a non-stick skillet on medium heat. Once heated, placed patty on and grill, flipping at half time.

Serve alongside a lettuce salad with vegetables and low-fat salad dressing.

NUTRITION FACTS

Serving Size: 2
Amount per serving
- Calories 324
- Total Fat 14g
- Total Carbs 34g
- Protein 55g

19. Lunch - Quinoa Carb Salad

A small and quick lunch jammed full of protein goodness.

INGREDIENTS

- 1 - cup Quinoa
- 1 - cup Soy Beans
- 1 - Red Bell Pepper
- 1/4 - cup chopped Coriander
- 1 - Lime
- 1 - tbsp Olive Oil
- 1/2 - tbsp each of Garlic Powder, Onion Powder, Cumin, and Paprika
- Salt and Pepper, to taste

Optional Add-ins

- 1/2 - cup cooked Black Beans
- 1/2 - chopped Red Onion
- 1 - chopped Tomato
- 1/2 - chopped Cucumber
- 1/4 - cup Hummus
- A dollop of Peanut Butter to increase healthy fats and protein

DIRECTIONS

Cook Quinoa for about 5 mins - depending how soft you like it could be up to 15minutes. Reduce to a simmer and cover. Remember Quinoa soaks up a lot of water so you may have to keep topping it up.

In a separate small saucepan, boil Soy Beans in water until fully cooked (check packaging) If you cook the beans the night before this makes it very quick

Once Quinoa and Soy beans are fully cooked, add all ingredients in a large bowl and mix until all flavors are combined.

NUTRITION FACTS

Serving Size Per serving, recipe makes 4 servings
Amount per serving

- Calories 141
- Total Fat 6g
- Total Carbs 16g
- Protein 12g

20. Lunch - Mushroom and Quinoa Stack

A Quorn and Quinoa punch that delivers a solid 18 grams of Vegetable Protein.

INGREDIENTS

- 2 - large Mushroom Portabella Caps rinsed clean and dried
- 1 - cup cooked Quinoa
- 1/2 - cup crumbled Tempeh OR Quorn Pieces
- 1/2 - Onion, diced
- 1 - cup Spinach
- 1 - Tomato, sliced
- 2 - tbsp grated Cheese OR fat-free Mozzarella
- 1 - tbsp Olive Oil
- 1/2 - tbsp each of Paprika, Cumin, Garlic Powder, and Onion Powder

Add Sea Salt and Black Pepper.

DIRECTIONS

Pre heat oven at 180C
Heat olive oil in a large pan over medium heat.
Add onion and Tempeh/Quorn to pan and sauté for 2-3 minutes, or until onion begins to soften.
Add Quinoa, spices, salt and pepper and sauté a few more minutes.
On a baking sheet, place Portobello mushrooms brushed lightly with olive oil.
Stack mushroom caps with spinach, Quinoa mixture, sliced tomatoes, and grated cheese.
Cook for 5 minutes in pre heated oven.

Tip - I often make double the portion and have this the next day.

NUTRITION

Serving Size: 2
Amount per serving
- Calories 324
- Total Fat 14g
- Total Carbs 34g
- Protein 18.25g

21. Lunch - Pasta with Peppers

Delicious 43 gram carb meal - perfect for a post-workout energy boost.

INGREDIENTS

- 1 - cup fresh sliced Mushrooms
- 3 - chopped Onions
- 1 - large Green Pepper - cut into strips
- 3 - cups uncooked Rigatoni - *go for gluten free*
- 1 - jar (24 oz.) chunky spaghetti sauce
- 1 - cup Shredded Italian Mozzarella-Parmesan Cheese Blend

DIRECTIONS

Heat oven to 190C. Sauté onions, peppers, and mushrooms for 5 minutes, or until cooked through. Meanwhile, cook pasta as directed on package. So really you want it soft, but not too soft!
Drain pasta and add pepper & mushroom mixture to baking dish with spaghetti sauce; stir. Bake 15 to 20 minutes until heated through. Top with cheese; bake 2 to 3 minutes or until melted.

NUTRITION FACTS

Servings 6
Amount Per Serving
- Calories: 282.2
- Total Fat: 7.3 g
- Total Carbs: 43 g
- Protein: 11.9 g

22. Lunch - Fat-free Stuffed Pasta Shells

The perfect lunch or snacks on the go - 4 shells = 23 grams of protein. Try Gluten free pasta and see how that goes down.

INGREDIENTS

- 12 - Jumbo Shell Pastas
- 110g - fat-free Cream Cheese
- 170g - fat-free Cottage Cheese
- 1 - cup fat-free shredded Mozzarella
- 1 - cup chopped Mushrooms
- 2 - cups Marinara sauce
- 3 - tsp granulated Garlic
- 1/2 - tbsp dried Oregano
- 1/2 - tbsp dried Parsley
- 1 - tsp dried Rosemary

DIRECTIONS

Pre heat oven to 180C.
Boil jumbo pasta shells in a saucepan until they are nearly done -- al dente.
Drain and rinse under cold water. Set aside.
Mix all the cream cheese, cottage cheese, mozzarella cheese, mushrooms and spices in a large bowl.
With a spoon - pack pasta shells with cheese mixture.
Place each stuffed pasta shell into an oven-safe high sided container.
Pour marinara evenly over stuffed shells.
Cover with foil and place into oven for about 20 minutes.

NUTRITION FACTS

Servings: 4
Amount Per Serving
- Calories: 281.0
- Total Fat: 1.7 g
- Total Carbs: 38.6 g
- Protein: 27.4 g

23. Dinner - Quorn Mince Lasagne

Who can resist a hearty helping of Quorn Lasagne at 19grams of protein?

INGREDIENTS

- 3 - Cups Quorn Mince
- 1 - Medium Onion
- 1 - tbsp Garlic powder
- 1 - tin Canned Tomatoes
- 1 - cup of Water
- 8 - Lasagne sheets
- 1 - tbsp Parsley
- 1 - tbsp Basil
- 1 - tbsp ground Oregano
- 1 - cup Fat free Cottage Cheese
- 0.25 - cup reduced fat grated Parmesan cheese
- 1 - cup Spaghetti Sauce

DIRECTIONS

Pre heat oven at 180C.
In a frying pan cook the Quorn mince following packets instructions.
Add onion, garlic, tomatoes and spaghetti sauce, Stir in parsley, basil, and oregano.
In oven-proof dish layer in Lasagne sheets and mince mixture.
Spread Cottage cheese over top layer and sprinkle grated Parmesan cheese on top.
Cook in oven for 20 minutes.

NUTRITION FACTS

Servings: 4
Amount Per Serving
- Calories: 290.9
- Total Fat: 5.0 g
- Total Carbs: 43.9 g
- Protein: 19.5 g

24. Dinner - Ricotta Cheese Lasagne

A twist on the Lasagne with delicious Ricotta Cheese delivering 40 grams of carbs and 20 grams of Protein.

INGREDIENTS

- 400g - of Ricotta Cheese
- 1 - Medium Onion
- 1 - tbsp Garlic powder
- 1 - tin Canned Tomatoes
- 1 - cup of Water
- 8 - Lasagne sheets
- 1 - tbsp Parsley
- 1 - tbsp Basil
- 1 - tbsp ground Oregano
- 0.25 - cup reduced fat grated Parmesan cheese
- 1 - cup Spaghetti Sauce

DIRECTIONS

Pre heat oven at 180C.
Mix all ingredients in a large bowl except Lasagne sheets.
In oven-proof dish layer in Lasagne sheets and above mixture.
Sprinkle grated Parmesan cheese on top.
Cook in oven for 20 minutes.

NUTRITION FACTS

Servings: 4
Amount Per Serving
- Calories: 290.9
- Total Fat:7.0 g
- Total Carbs: 43.9 g
- Protein: 20.5 g

25. Dinner - Tofu Chilli and Quinoa

A two-serving beast at 27 grams of protein per serving.

INGREDIENTS

- 1 - cup Quinoa
- 1/4 - cup Brown sugar
- 1/4 -cup Soy sauce
- 1 - tsp Chili sauce
- 2 - tsp Sesame oil
- 2 - minced garlic cloves
- 1 - tsp grated fresh ginger
- Pinch of sea salt
- 340g - Tofu
- 1 - tsp olive oil

DIRECTIONS

Cook Quinoa as directed on the packet.
Mix brown sugar, soy sauce, chili sauce, sesame oil, garlic cloves, ginger and sea salt in a small bowl and set aside.

Pour olive oil into sauce pan and heat.
Fry Tofu in pan for about 10 minutes.
Pour sauce into pan and cook for 3-5 minutes. Sauce will thicken and the Tofu will absorb most of it.

Then add to Quinoa and mix thoroughly - allow to simmer for 5 minutes while stirring. Then it's ready to serve.

NUTRITION FACTS

Serves 2
Amount per serving
- Calories 329
- Total Fat 18 g
- Total Carbs 27 g
- Protein 27 g

26. Dinner - Macaroni Cheese

Simple pasta dish that tastes great and provides 45 grams of carbs and 19 grams of protein.

INGREDIENTS

- 220g - of pasta of choice
- 1/2 - cup milk (OR unflavored Coconut/Rice/Soya milk etc)
- 1/4 - cup unflavoured Pea Protein Powder
- 1/4 - cup grated Cheddar Cheese
- 1 - tbsp coconut flour
- 1 - tsp of Parmesan Cheese
- Garlic salt to taste
- Italian seasoning
- Dry Parsley OR Basil

DIRECTIONS

Cook the pasta of your choice until al dente.
Mix all of the milk, Pea Protein, Cheddar Cheese, Coconut Flour into a saucepan. Bring sauce to a simmer and continue to stir until all of the components are well combined and sauce thickens.
Drain water from pasta.
Add the sauce to your pasta, mix and simmer for 5 minutes stirring occasionally.

Serve and sprinkle with Parmesan cheese - absolutely perfect!

NUTRITION FACTS

Serving size: 4
Amount per serving
- Calories 271
- Total Fat 4 g
- Total Carbs 45 g
- Protein 19 g

27. Dinner - Hot Tofu and Rice

Spicy Tofu delivers an impressive 18 grams of protein.

INGREDIENTS

- 1 - package extra firm Tofu
- 2 - cups cooked Brown Rice
- 2 - tbsp Low-sodium Soy sauce
- 1 - tsp each of Ginger, Garlic Powder, and Onion Powder
- 1 - tsp Chili Paste
- 1 - bunch chopped Broccoli
- 1 - sliced Red Bell Pepper
- 1 - sliced Orange Bell Pepper

DIRECTIONS

Chop tofu into cubes.
Cook brown rice in a sauce pan of boiling water following packet instructions.
In a large sauce pan heat olive oil over medium heat.
Add broccoli and bell pepper and stir until lightly softened.

Heat another pan to medium heat and add Tofu.
Cook tofu for 5 minutes, stirring occasionally until all sides get cooked.

Serve brown rice and top with tofu, veggies, and green onions.

NUTRITION FACTS

Serving: 4
Amount per serving
- Calories 257
- Total Fat 8g
- Total Carbs 13g
- Protein 18g

28. Dinner - Cashew Chicken

Cashew chicken is a favourite among muscle-builders because it provides two quality types of protein. Cashews contain plenty of iron, zinc, and trace minerals.

INGREDIENTS

- 1 lb. of chicken, sliced
- ½ cup of cashews
- ¼ cup soy sauce
- 1/8 cup peanut sauce
- Wheat noodles
- Vegetables
- Sesame oil

DIRECTIONS

Start by heating up your wok or skillet to 300 degrees or low/medium heat. Pour 1 tbsp. of sesame oil into the pan or use butter if you don't have any. Cook the chicken first. Wait until it is cooked through before adding your choice of vegetables. Any green veggies, such as broccoli, seaweed, or veggies like carrots should be used. Onions and bell peppers are also filled with appropriate nutrients for skin health. Cook the veggies until they are soft.

You can also add in the soy sauce and peanut sauce to help steam the veggies. Cook the noodles per package instructions. Once all is cooked, add in the cashews, mix it up and serve.

NUTRITION FACTS

Serving size: 1 bowl
Amount per serving
- Calories 492
- Total Fat 26 g
- Total Carbs 38 g
- Protein 32 g

29. Dinner - Pork with Apricot Sauce

Apricots are very healthy and go for lean pork roast or pork chop to keep the cholesterol down.

INGREDIENTS

- 1 lb. pork
- ¼ cup Dijon
- ¼ cup apricot jelly or fresh apricots
- 1 onion
- ½ cup vegetable or chicken broth

In a skillet, put the vegetable broth, and onion in and place the pork into the pan. Cook one side. After you turn the pork over, dump the Dijon mustard and apricot mixture into the skillet. If you use fresh apricots, they need to be cut into chunks and the juice squeezed into the pan. Cook until the other side of the pork is nicely cooked. It takes about 20 minutes. Serve with the sauce to help keep the pork moist.

NUTRITION FACTS

Serving size: 1 bowl
Amount per serving
- Calories 392
- Total Fat 20 g
- Total Carbs 26 g
- Protein 28 g

30. Dinner – Beef and Broccoli Powerhouse

Combine protein-rich red meat with heart-healthy broccoli and antioxidant-packed blackberries.

Blackberries adds an extra tang of flavor along with free-radical fighting antioxidants, while the high-protein combo of beef and broccoli means you'll be making gains while getting good-for-you vitamins and minerals.

Sesame oil, ginger, and garlic - All three are known to be great for heart health!

<u>INGREDIENTS</u>

- Lean Flank Steak, Thinly Sliced 1-1/2 Lbs.
- Broccoli Florets, Raw 3 Cups
- Red Bell Pepper, Sliced 1
- Yellow Bell Pepper, Sliced 1
- Sauce Ingredients
- Low-Sodium Beef Stock 1/2 Cup
- Liquid Aminos Or Low-Sodium Soy Sauce 1/2 Cup
- Blackberries 1 Cup
- Garlic, Minced Or Paste 1 Tbsp
- Ginger 1 Tbsp
- Sesame Oil 1 Tbsp
- Arrowroot Starch 2 Tbsp
- Rice Vinegar 1 1/2 Tbsp
- Organic Raw Honey 3 Tbsp (Optional)
- Garnish Ingredients
- Green Onions
- Sesame Seeds

DIRECTIONS

In a small bowl, whisk together beef stock, liquid aminos, ginger, sesame oil, arrowroot starch, and rice wine vinegar.

Set a saucepan or small skillet on medium-high heat, and spray it with a little olive oil. Once the pan is hot, toss in garlic and blackberries. Sauté the blackberries for about 6-8 minutes, allowing them to explode under the heat. Using a spatula, gently mash down the berries, continuously stirring them so they don't burn.

Add the bowl of sauce to the skillet. Reduce the heat to medium, and stir the sauce so it begins to thicken. If you want the sauce to be sweeter, add organic raw honey, and stir. Once the sauce is smooth, remove it from the heat and set it aside.

Set a stir-fry wok or large nonstick skillet on medium-high heat. Once the wok is hot, toss in thin slices of beef and cook for about 4 minutes, or until the majority of the beef is no longer pink.

Add diced bell peppers to the skillet, and stir quickly. Try to sear the bell peppers. Cook for about 3 minutes, then add the broccoli florets.

Tip: If you prefer to have a sear on the veggies, remove the beef from the skillet before adding in the greens. Once the veggies are seared, add the beef back to the skillet.

Cook the beef and broccoli together for about 5 minutes, and continue to stir with a spatula. Reduce the heat to medium, and pour in the sauce. Stir the mixture or shake and toss the food in the wok to ensure the stir fry is evenly coated in the sauce. Cook and stir for another 2-3 minutes.

Garnish with green onions and sesame seeds. Enjoy the stir fry with a serving of brown rice or quinoa.

NUTRITION FACTS

Serving size: 1 bowl
Recipe yields: 4 serving
Amount per serving
- Calories 392
- Total Fat 14 g
- Total Carbs 26 g
- Protein 40 g

31. Dinner - Mango Chicken With Coconut Cauliflower Rice

This simple-to-make, low-carb mango chicken is served over coconut cauliflower rice. With a little fresh ginger and habanero, it packs a delicious punch!

INGREDIENTS

- 2.5 tsp coconut oil
- 1.5 tsp fresh ginger, minced
- 1 tsp garlic, minced
- 1/2 tsp habanero pepper, minced (optional)
- 3/4 cup 100% orange mango juice
- 1/2 tbsp coconut aminos
- 1 tsp tapioca flour

CHICKEN INGREDIENTS

- 3 tbsp tapioca flour
- 8 oz chicken breast
- 2 tbsp coconut oil
- salt, to taste
- pepper, to taste

CAULIFLOWER RICE INGREDIENTS

- 3 cups cauliflower
- 2 tsp coconut oil
- 2 tbsp unsweetened coconut flakes

GARNISH INGREDIENTS

- 1/2 large mango, cubed
- cilantro to taste, roughly chopped
- green onion to taste, roughly chopped

- 1 tsp sesame seeds

SAUCE DIRECTIONS

Heat 1-1/2 teaspoons of coconut oil in a large skillet over medium heat.

Add in the ginger, garlic, and habanero pepper, and cook until fragrant, about 1 minute. Add in the juice and coconut aminos. Raise the temperature to high heat, and bring to a boil. While liquid is boiling, place the tapioca flour in a small bowl.
Once the liquid comes to a boil, add 2 teaspoons of it to the bowl with the tapioca flour and whisk until smooth. While stirring constantly, pour the tapioca mixture into the sauce and boil for 2 minutes.
After the sauce has boiled, reduce the heat to medium-low and simmer, stirring frequently, until the sauce reduces by about 1/4 and becomes shiny, about 6-7 minutes.
Transfer sauce to a large bowl to let it cool and thicken while you make the chicken.

CHICKEN INSTRUCTIONS

Place the tapioca flour in a large Ziploc bag. Cut the chicken into cubes, season it with salt and pepper and add it into the bag, shaking until evenly coated in the flour.
In a medium pan, heat 1 tablespoon of the coconut oil over medium-high heat. Place half of the chicken into the pan, being careful not to crowd it, and cook until golden and browned, about 2-3 minutes. Flip and repeat.
Transfer the chicken to a paper-towel-lined plate, and blot off any excess oil. Repeat with the remaining chicken. If the chicken starts cooking too quickly, turn the heat down slightly.

While the chicken cooks, place the cauliflower in a large food processor and process until broken down and rice-like.

Heat the 2 teaspoons of coconut oil in a large pan over medium-high heat and add the cauliflower and coconut flakes. Cook until lightly golden, about 2-3 minutes. Cover, reduce the heat to medium, and cook until the cauliflower is tender, about 2-4 minutes.
Transfer the chicken and mango cubes into the bowl with the sauce and toss until evenly coated.
Divide the chicken and cauliflower between two plates and garnish with cilantro, green onion and sesame seeds.

NUTRITION FACTS

Serving size: 1 bowl
Recipe yields: 2 bowls
- Calories: 591
- Fat: 31 g
- Carbs: 43 g
- Protein: 36 g

32. Dinner - Orange Beef Stir-Fry Sweet Potato Noodles And Kale

In 30 minutes and this orange beef stir-fry packed with healthy carbs and muscle-bulging protein can be on your plate.

STIR-FRY INGREDIENTS

- 1 large sweet potato
- 2.5 tsp coconut oil
- 1 tsp fresh ginger, minced
- 0.5 lb top sirloin steak, cut into bite-sized pieces

SAUCE INGREDIENTS

- 1 cup 100% orange juice
- 2 tsp fresh ginger, minced
- 1 tbsp + 1 tsp coconut aminos
- 1 tbsp + 1 tsp honey
- 6-8 cups kale
- salt and pepper, to taste

DIRECTIONS

Spiralize the sweet potato using the 3-millimeter-blade spiralizer.
Heat 1-1/2 teaspoons of the coconut oil in a large pan over medium heat. Add in the potato noodles and cook until they just begin to soften, about 5-7 minutes. Place into a bowl and cover to keep warm.
Heat the remaining teaspoon of oil in the pan over medium heat, and add in 1 teaspoon of fresh ginger. Cook until the ginger is lightly browned and fragrant, about 1 minute.

Add the steak and cook until it reaches desired doneness. Drain the fat and place into a bowl. Cover it to keep warm, and set aside.

In a small bowl, whisk together all the sauce ingredients except the kale and toss into the pan. Turn the heat up to high, and boil the sauce until it just begins to thicken, about 2-3 minutes.

Turn the heat down to medium and toss in the kale. Cook until the kale begins to wilt.
Divide the noodles and steak between two dishes and top with the sauce and kale mixture.

NUTRITION FACTS

Serving size: 1/2 recipe
Recipe yields: 2 servings
- Calories: 546
- Fat: 12 g
- Carbs: 65 g
- Protein: 38 g

33. Dinner - Cheddar-Stuffed Burgers

You can't go wrong with a burger and Cheddar Cheese! Burgers are a big weakness of mine, and home-made you just have to say yes please.

INGREDIENTS

- Ground Beef (80/20): 2 Lbs.
- Sharp Cheddar Cheese: 8 Oz.
- Olive Oil: 1/2 Cup
- Iceberg Lettuce: 8 Large Leaves
- Medium Tomato: 1
- Worcestershire Sauce: 2-1/2 Tbsp
- Haas Avocado: 1
- Dill Pickle Spears
- Salt And Pepper: To Taste

DIRECTIONS

Combine meat, Worcestershire sauce, salt, and pepper to taste in a medium bowl. Blend well.
Divide meat into 8 equal portions and shape each into a ball.

Poke a deep hole in each ball and fill with 1 ounce of cheese. Mold meat around cheese to enclose, and flatten each burger to a 3/4-inch-thick patty.

Cook each burger in olive oil to desired doneness, about 5 minutes per side for medium.

Top each burger with avocado, a slice of tomato, and a pickle spear, and wrap in a lettuce leaf.

NUTRITION FACTS

Serving size: 1 burger
Recipe yields: 8 servings
Amount per serving:
- Calories 585
- Fat 46 g
- Carbs 4 g
- Protein 38 g

34. Snack - Mexican Black Beans and Avocado

Perfect pre-workout snack giving you a hefty 40 grams of carbs.

INGREDIENTS

- 1/2 - cup cooked Brown Rice
- 1/3 - cup cooked Black Beans
- 2 - heaping spoonful's of Salsa
- 1/4 - sliced Avocado
- 2 - tbsp plain Fat-free Greek Yogurt

A hot sauce of your choosing or something like Sweet and Sour - just a dash.

DIRECTIONS

This is ideal if you have ingredients left over. Mix all ingredients in a large bowl - serve and enjoy.

NUTRITION

Serving Size 1
Amount per serving
- Calories 292
- Total Fat 9g
- Total Carbs 40g
- Protein 12g

35. Snack - Raisin Oatmeal Cookie

Did someone say cookies?

INGREDIENTS

- 1/2 - cup Rolled Oats
- 1 - Egg
- 11 g - of Unsweetened Applesauce
- 14 g - Raisins
- 1 - Tbsp Cinnamon
- 1 - Tbsp Stevia

DIRECTIONS

Preheat oven to 350.
Combine all the ingredients in a small bowl.
Pour into pre-sprayed Ramekins (small over-proof dish).
Place the Ramekins in the oven for 20 minutes, or until the oats are slightly toasted.

NUTRITION

Recipe serves 2
Amount per serving
- Calories 185
- Total Fat 4 g
- Total Carb 38 g
- Protein 6.6 g

36. Snack - Fast Yogurt and Apricot

A top-notch evening snack before bed to see you through the night with slow proteins and fats.

INGREDIENTS

- 220 g - of Greek Style Yogurt
- 1-2 - palm-fulls of raw or roasted Almonds (unsalted and unsweetened)
- 1 - palm-full of dried Apricot
- 1 - packet of Stevia (zero calorie sweetener) or a bit of agave or Honey

DIRECTIONS

Mix all the above ingredients in a large bowl - serve in a small bowl and eat up!

NUTRITION FACTS

Serving Size 1
Amount per serving
- Calories 428
- Total Fat 23g
- Total Carbs 31g
- Protein 23g

37. Snack - Protein Banana Smoothie

A stunning protein shake delivering 32 grams of protein.

INGREDIENTS

- 500ml - of Water
- 1 - Scoop of Rice Protein
- 1/2 - Scoop of Pea Protein
- 2 - Bananas
- 0.5 - cup skim milk (OR almond, soy, coconut, or cashew milk)
- 10 - Almonds
- 1 - Handful of Ice

DIRECTIONS

Add all the ingredients to a Blender and mix for 4 minutes. Pour into a shaker for on the go or a tall glass.

Tip - Don't neglect the ice - this really adds to the taste and density.

NUTRITION FACTS

Serving size: 1 shake
Amount per serving
- Calories 320
- Total Fat 8 g
- Total Carbs 32 g
- Protein 32 g

38. Snack - Guacamole Hummus

A great little dish giving you 22 grams of carbs - ideal with a protein shake.

INGREDIENTS

- 1 - can Chickpeas
- 1 - Avocado
- 1 - Jalapeano
- 1/4 - cup chopped cilantro
- Juice from 1 Lime

DIRECTIONS

Mix ingredients together in a large bowl until thoroughly mixed.
Then serve with vegetables, pita chips, or snack of your choice.

Combine with one of the smoothies for more of a protein hit.

NUTRITION FACTS

Serves 4
Amount per serving
- Calories 200
- Total Fat 9 g
- Total Carbs 22 g
- Protein 7.5g

39. Snack - Sweet Cinnamon Quinoa Punch

Walnuts and Quinoa mix to give you a 12grams of protein and 29 grams of carbs.

INGREDIENTS

- 1/4 - cup Quinoa
- 1 - palm-full of Walnuts or Pecans 7-10 individual nuts)
- 1 - palm-full of Blackberries or Blueberries
- Sprinkle of Cinnamon

Sweeten with Stevia (zero-calorie, natural sweetener) or use agave nectar or Honey

DIRECTIONS

Cook your Quinoa in a sauce pan as per instructions on packet. Drain once cooked.
Add the walnuts, blackberries, cinnamon and Stevia and mix it all together with a spoon. Serve hot!

NUTRITION FACTS

Serving Size 1
Amount per serving
- Calories 418
- Total Fat 26g
- Total Carbs 29g
- Protein 12g

40. Snack - Protein Apple and Celery Smoothie

The super shake - 32 grams of protein and 32 grams of carbs - no messing around here.

INGREDIENTS

- 500ml - of Water
- 1 - Scoop of Rice Protein
- 1/2 - Scoop of Pea Protein
- 1 - apple
- 2 - Sticks of Celery
- 0.5 - Cup of skim milk (OR almond, soy, coconut, or cashew milk)
- 10 - Almonds
- 1 - Handful of Ice

DIRECTIONS

Add all the ingredients to a Blender and mix for 4 minutes. Pour into Shaker for on the go or a tall glass.

Tip - Add the ice – it really helps. You could also add a dollop of peanut butter instead of the almonds if you preferred.

NUTRITION FACTS

Serving size: 1 shake
Amount per serving
- Calories 320
- Total Fat 8 g
- Total Carbs 32 g
- Protein 32 g

41. Snack - Peppermint Oatmeal Shake

INGREDIENTS

- 2 scoops chocolate protein
- 1 cup sugar-free vanilla ice cream
- 1 cup oatmeal
- 2 cups nonfat milk
- 1/2 cup water
- 1/2 tsp peppermint extract

DIRECTIONS

Mix all the ingredients together in a blender – and serve!
Simple as!

NUTRITION FACTS

Serving size: 1 shake
Amount per serving
- Calories 340
- Total Fat 8 g
- Total Carbs 30 g
- Protein 48 g

42. Snack - Iced Breakfast Shake

Blending whey protein and instant breakfast packs a dual carb and protein hit.

INGREDIENTS

- 1 cup skim milk
- 1 scoop whey protein
- 2 tsp safflower oil
- 1 handful ice
- 1 banana
- 1 package instant breakfast

DIRECTIONS

Mix all the ingredients together in a blender – and serve! Simple as!

NUTRITION

Serving size: 1 shake
Amount per serving
- Calories 270
- Total Fat 12 g
- Total Carbs 30 g
- Protein 28 g

43. Snack - Almond Blast Shake

This protein shake is a brilliant post-workout recovery drink, delivering a solid 58 grams of protein.

INGREDIENTS

- 2 scoops vanilla whey protein
- 1-1/2 cups skim milk
- 1/2 cup dry oatmeal
- 1/2 cup raisins
- 12 slivered almonds
- 1 tbsp peanut butter

DIRECTIONS

Mix all the ingredients together in a blender – and serve! Simple as!

NUTRITION FACTS

Serving size: 1 shake
Amount per serving
- Calories 470
- Total Fat 12 g
- Total Carbs 45 g
- Protein 58 g

44. Snack – The Berry Super Shake

This shake is packed with protein, fibre, healthy fats and probiotics.

INGREDIENTS

- 12 oz water
- 1 cup spinach
- 2 cups frozen mixed berries
- 1/2 cup plain low-fat yogurt
- 2 scoops vanilla protein powder
- 1 tbsp walnuts
- 1 tbsp ground flaxseed

DIRECTIONS

Mix all the ingredients together in a blender – and serve! Simple as!

NUTRITION FACTS

Serving size: 1 shake
Amount per serving
- Calories 500
- Total Fat 11 g
- Total Carbs 54 g
- Protein 57 g

45. Snack – Chocolate And Banana Shake

You'd never guess that a cup of spinach is hiding in this delicious chocolate and peanut butter shake.

INGREDIENTS

1. 12 oz water, milk, or yogurt
2. 2 scoops chocolate flavored protein powder
3. 1 banana
4. 1 cup of spinach
5. 2 tbsp of natural peanut butter
6. 1 tbsp cacao nibs or dark cocoa powder

DIRECTIONS

Mix all the ingredients together in a blender – and serve!

NUTRITION

Serving size: 1 shake
Amount per serving
- Calories 585
- Total Fat 22 g
- Total Carbs 38 g
- Protein 59 g

46. Shake - Chocolate Cherry Shake

INGREDIENTS

- 12 oz water, milk, or yogurt
- 2 scoops chocolate flavored protein powder
- 2 cups of sweet dark cherries, pits removed
- 1 cups of spinach
- 1 tbsp of walnuts
- 1 tbsp ground flax
- 1 tbsp cacao nibs or dark cocoa powder

DIRECTIONS

Mix all the ingredients together in a blender – and serve!
Simple as!

NUTRITION FACTS

Serving size: 1 shake
Amount per serving
- Calories 530
- Total Fat 13 g
- Total Carbs 47 g
- Protein 56 g

47. Snack - Superfood Shake

Deeply colored fruits and vegetables like beets and cherries and jammed with healthy nutrients that can boost athletic performance and help muscle recovery.

INGREDIENTS

- 1/2 cup frozen cherries
- 8 oz water
- 1/2 cup chopped raw beets
- 1/2 cup frozen strawberries
- 1/2 cup frozen blueberries
- 1/2 banana
- 1 scoop chocolate whey protein
- 1 tbsp ground flaxseed

DIRECTIONS

Mix all the ingredients together in a blender – and serve! Simple as!

NUTRITION FACTS

Serving size: 1 shake
Amount per serving
- Calories 329
- Total Fat 4 g
- Total Carbs 52 g
- Protein 28 g

48. Snack – The Power Shake

This shake packs 33 grams of healthy protein.

INGREDIENTS

- ¼ cup low fat cottage cheese
- 1 cup blueberries (fresh or frozen)
- 1 scoop vanilla protein powder
- 2 tbsp flaxseed meal
- 2 tbsp walnuts, chopped
- 1½ cups water
- 3 ice cubes

DIRECTIONS

Mix all the ingredients together in a blender – and serve!

NUTRITION FACTS

Serving size: 1 shake
Amount per serving
- Calories 389
- Total Fat 17 g
- Total Carbs 34 g
- Protein 33 g

49. Snacks – Choco Peanut Butter Smoothie

Drink this for the perfect afternoon snack. It's packed with protein, fibre, and antioxidants and peanuts!

INGREDIENTS

- Water as needed
- 2 tbsp flaxmeal
- 1 tbsp unsweetened cocoa powder
- 1 tbsp natural peanut butter
- 1 scoop chocolate whey protein powder

DIRECTIONS

Mix all the ingredients together in a blender – and serve!

NUTRITION FACTS

Serving size: 1 shake
Amount per serving
- Calories 347
- Total Fat 17 g
- Total Carbs 19 g
- Protein 33 g

50. Snack - Mango Shake

53 grams - A high calorie, high impact shake ideal for post or pre workout when you've really killed it with the weights.

INGREDIENTS

- 2 scoops vanilla whey protein powder
- 1 cup frozen chopped mango
- 1 oz of walnuts
- 12 oz orange juice
- Ice as needed

DIRECTIONS

Mix all the ingredients together in a blender – and serve!

NUTRITION FACTS

Serving size: 1 shake
Amount per serving
- Calories 700
- Total Fat 20 g
- Total Carbs 74 g
- Protein 53 g

Bonus - Snack - Summertime Blast

A bonus shake which is high carb hit to replenish lost energy jam-packed with healthy fruits and high vitamin C.

INGREDIENTS

- 2/3 cup seedless watermelon
- 1 scoop of Vanilla Isolate Whey
- 2 tsp lemon juice
- 1/2 cantaloupe
- 1 banana
- 1/4 cup pineapple
- 2/3 cup ice
- 4 to 5 fresh basil leaves

DIRECTIONS

Mix all the ingredients together in a blender – and serve!

NUTRITION

Serving size: 1 shake
Amount per serving
- Calories 182
- Total Fat 1 g
- Total Carbs 47 g
- Protein 28 g

To Kill it – Maximising Gains

So what is the number one way to kill it...or in other words to make gains fast I hear you cry? It's very simple – Dietary Preparation.

One of the biggest mistakes people make is not planning ahead and this is crucial to building muscle mass. Letting your body go without quality fuel will stunt your progress if not completely stop it. There really is no point hammering away in the gym to not provide your body with the right nutrients to grow.

Some nutritionists say following a solid diet is 50% of building size, others rate it as high as 90%! Yes 90% of what you look like is down to diet, and 10% weight training. I'd personally say it's more of a 40% training, 60% diet. It's too easy to eat junk after training and use the training to justify it. If we want to build a quality physique, we must be prepared to go all the way.

How much protein do you need?

The RDA is 0.8 grams per kilogram of lean bodyweight (U.S. Food and Nutrition Board, 1980) for sedentary adults (1 kilogram=2.2 pounds)
However you should be aiming for 1.5- 2.4 grams of protein per kilogram of bodyweight. More towards the 2.4 grams will have a maximal effect on building muscle. So weigh yourself and work out now what you should be consuming.

Many of the bodybuilders, trainers, and nutritionists agree on these rough figures. Ultimately you will need to find out how your body responds to more protein.

Let's move on to tactics for preparation.

The Big Shop

Firstly you can do a big shop on a Sunday and buy enough food to last until the following Sunday. How much exactly will depend on your nutritional needs. But I'd look at these meals and buy a fair amount and probably more than you need. Once you've done a few shops you'll know exactly what you need. Then you can prepare meals on the Sunday for the next few days so you're not caught short.

3 Day Shop

Another way is to buy enough food to last from Sunday until Wednesday and prepare meals for all those days on the Sunday. Then on the Wednesday I would plan and buy ingredients for Thursday through to Sunday. You will then never find yourself short of key foods to help keep your macro-nutrients at optimal level. Once you've done this a few times it will become second nature and you'll always have the right food to hand.

Something I do now is buy all my fruit and vegetables from the local market. Firstly the prices are much cheaper, and more importantly the quality is superb. It's all fresh and delicious. Plus if you eat eggs you can buy those too from a farmer.

Ordering online means you can purchase most of your food and get it delivered with ease.

So that's the end of my book! I just wanted to thank you for checking out my book and i hope you enjoy the recipes here. Please give my book a review, it really helps me and allows me to continue to write useful content for building muscle.

These recipes are guides for you to experiment with. More importantly I hope they help you with your muscle building gains and while aiding a healthy lifestyle.

-M

How To Build The Rugby Player Body
Hardcover
https://www.createspace.com/6252083

KDP
https://www.amazon.com/dp/B0187UJS34